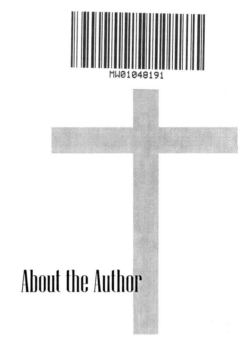

About the Author

Dr. Steven B. DavidSon is founder of the National Association of Certified Christ-based Counselors in its 12th year. He designed the Christ-based Counseling model, but refers to Jesus as the origin, architect, and empowerment of the Christ-based Counseling framework. Thousands have taken advantage of his works in areas such as marriage, homosexuality, depression, anorexia and bulimia, child discipline, and addiction just to name a few. His Christ-based model is far superior to Christian counseling where often psychology is employed under the guise of sprinkled Scripture text. Dr. Paul Carlin the director and founder of Therapon Institute calls Dr. DavidSon's works the most profound Christ-based concepts he has ever witnessed.

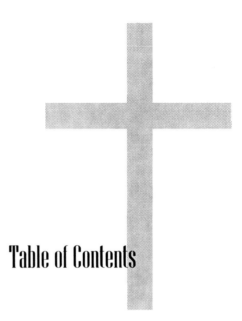

Table of Contents

Christ-based Counseling Preparation and Distinction

Christ-based Counseling (CBC) Preparation and Distinction

Persons who are reading this book are seeking wholeness for one's self or others. There are three functional investments counselees or other participants must make in Christ-based Counseling exercises. The participant must:

- ✓ READ
- ✓ RESPOND
- ✓ REITERATE

This means the counselee reads the information, answers each question, and discusses or shares the answers with another person. The questions are divided into blocks of fifty questions each session. The participant can be any person interested in the process (e.g., minister, counselor, friend, relative, etc.).

Whether it is used with or without a Christ-based Counselor, the most effective use of the Christ-based Counseling approach is to begin with the Process of Being Made Whole. I strongly recommend that participants complete the Process of Being Made Whole (PBMW) as a prerequisite to the specific counseling needed.

The Process of Being Made Whole, and accompanying course is on the internet at Christbasedcounseling.org. Simply click-on the link or door for the School of Counseling and Certification, and scroll down to The Process of Being Made Whole link. Print out the on-line guide. Use the guide to answer the questions in the on-line course. This on-line course link is the next link beneath the Process of Being Made Whole link.

The Process of Being Made Whole and questions are also included in this book for your convenience. Both the guide and questions are a mirror image of the web versions. If you have completed the Process of Being Made Whole previously, and you have mastered all seven constituents, this will be an excellent refresher.

Christ-based Counseling's Distinction

I have counseled literally hundreds of couples and individuals. Unlike the psychological and medical professions, I assure counselees there will be positive change in forty-five days. Persons who meticulously follow each step and who stay-the-course over time may not resolve the issues they face in forty-five days, but there will be change. They will establish significant progress toward the wholeness they seek. This is because the principles in Christ-based Counseling operate in the angelic realm where the most effective powers and authorities operate to change the physical realm.

Christ-based Counseling is also distinguished from Christian counseling or Christian psychology where the basis is often psychotherapy under the guise of sprinkled Scripture text. Christ-based Counseling is based on a sound Biblical system where the whole approach is thoroughly Biblical.

Finally, this is not a novel, motivational guide, or academic text. This approach is a spiritually empowered process with principles the believer must observe for a lifetime. Typically, the behavior and habits we desire to overcome have been with us for years. Therefore, it may be necessary to review the Christ-based Counseling principles numerous times.

PART I

Understanding the Problem and Root Cause, A Christ-based Counseling Perspective

Understanding the Problem and Root Cause, A Christ-based Counseling Perspective

Eating Ourselves to Death

The Centers for Disease Control reports that obesity is a national epidemic. Based on the Year 2000 data, more than sixty percent of the adult population is overweight or obese. Annually, more than three-hundred fifty thousand (350,000) deaths are attributed to obesity. The prevalence of overweight children is also climbing at an alarming rate. Food consumption is a causative factor along with portions and content[1].

I was inspired to focus on this topic by a personal experience. I was "encouraged" to fast. It was simply placed in my spirit to fast for seven days. This inner voice was affirmed by two persons. Although I fast systematically half-days every Saturday and Sunday, the results of fasting seven days was dramatic.

I noticed a number of physical differences. First, there was noticeable weight loss. Secondly, the experience represented a physical cleansing. Gases and other toxins passed through my body.

---

[1] Centers for Disease Control Web Site, CDC.gov/NCCDPHP/DNPA/OBESITY/ "This is under review"

Some physical problems were eliminated, which improved other bodily functions. Thirdly, there was something uniquely spiritual about it. I can only describe it as a spiritually enhanced focus. Finally, my resounding conclusion was that I consume too much food. This experience launched this initiative and discovery of some fascinating Biblical principles rarely disclosed.

While there are many causes and dispositions one may assume during a fast, Jesus' fast was not typical. Jesus directed believers to maintain their typical daily functions and disposition. Clearly, this is what Jesus meant when He instructed His disciples not to fast as hypocrites (Matthew 6:16). This, "Christ-based" fast was not a sad and depressing experience for public recognition. This was uniquely different from the traditional fast, and the first hint that something else is at work with the Christ-based fast. In addition, the findings in this book demonstrate that fasting was not merely an instrument for spiritual pursuits.

There are volumes of literature and programs describing what a person must do for weight management. Most weight management programs focus on food intake or diet, and exercise. Stated simply, weight management involves calories-in and calories-out. The truth is that if a person does not dramatically reduce caloric consumption, there will be minimal weight loss success. There are plenty of diet programs available. Therefore, the real key is not an external-based eating program such as a diet. Furthermore, we must remember that weight management also involves persons who face, "weight deficit disorders" (e.g., Anorexia, Bulimia, etc.). Whatever the case, most people need internal empowerment for the results they desire.

This book reveals an important factor often neglected. There is a spiritual component to weight management, and there was much more in the life of Jesus concerning consumption control than fasting. This book shares principles from the very beginning of humanity. Jesus demonstrated these principles. This book provides the origin, rationale, and power sustaining the discipline He demonstrated in this area of His life. Furthermore, this is not a theoretical book. A host of people have observed the truths, employed the principles, and experienced the astonishing results. Thus, our trademarked theme, "Christ-based Weight Management, We Don't Diet, We Live By It (Him), The Living Bread."

Traditional Fasting

Many articles and books have been written on Biblical fasting. These cover the full scope of fasting including:

- ✓ Length of fast
- ✓ What to do while fasting
- ✓ Occasions to fast
- ✓ Types of fast
- ✓ Purposes for fasting

Those persons who have conducted Biblical research usually find common ground on all of the topics in the aforementioned.

Most writers agree the first place fasting is found is when Moses receives the Law (Exodus 34:28, Deuteronomy 9:9, 18). The duration of the fast is forty days. Elijah and Jesus also fasted for forty day periods (I Kings 19:18, Matthew 4:2). The fact that we are introduced to fasting when the Law is given to Moses has significance concerning fasting. I refer to this as a Mosaic fast representing a period when the Hebrews are transitioning into a new phase in their relationship with God. I will return to this fact later.

Most writers further agree that fasting is always done with a spiritual goal or purpose in mind. Therefore, most of them frown at the use of fasting for any other purpose. They argue that fasting should be done for "spiritual" purposes.

Simultaneously, the same writers use illustrations where some dire "physical" condition existed, which caused the person to pray and fast. No issue in the believer's life is purely spiritual and spiritual alone. Prayer is not a purely spiritual act. Faith is not a purely spiritual act. God's Word, while spiritual is not only given to spiritual manifestations. These are examples of spiritual instruments, which affect our material or "physical" circumstances.

People pray and exhibit faith because they typically desire some physical manifestation of what they pray for in the spiritual realm. The majority of spiritual virtues have physical or material representations.

People pray for families, jobs, houses, careers, ministries, and any other area of the human experience. However, when it comes to fasting there are those who believe that it must be a spiritual purpose.

Therefore, there needs to be clarity. Fasting can be used as a spiritual vehicle to a physical request, which is in the will of God. Persons can fast and pray for the same thing.

As shown above, there are several reasons for fasting, and this book identifies some profound findings about fasting.

The Genesis of Fasting

When I first began the Biblical research for this book, it was startling to discover that fasting does not appear in the Book of Genesis. Biblically, fasting is not apparent until the life of Moses. However, I believe the beginning or principal cause for fasting can be found in Genesis.

One has to look no further than the infamous Chapter 3 of Genesis. Rarely do we recognize that a major theme of this chapter is food consumption or eating. Beginning with the first verse, eating is referenced about sixteen times in the first nineteen verses.

Additionally, there is information, which suggests that food by definition is cursed:

> *Then to Adam He said, Because you have listened to the voice of your wife, and have eaten from the tree about which I commanded you, saying, 'You shall not eat from it'; Cursed is the ground because of you; In toil you shall eat of it all the days of your life. Both thorns and thistles it shall grow for you; And you shall eat the plants of the field; By the sweat of your face You shall eat bread, Till you return to the ground, Because from it you were taken; For you are dust, And to dust you shall return.*
> *(Gen. 3:17-19, NASB)*

Since man ate the forbidden fruit, the ground becomes cursed. Likewise, it is reasonable that everything proceeding from the ground is cursed. The result of this curse represents outcomes, which are undesirable including thorns and thistles. Contaminated plant life and bread are also a result of the curse. Sometimes bread is used generically representing all manner of sustenance (Leviticus 26:26, Psalms 105:16, Isaiah 3:1, etc.). However, it appears that bread, which comes forth from plant life is likely the object (i.e., wheat, rice, corn, etc.). Here is a translation of the cursed passages of the same text:

*The ground is cursed because of your act. Now, you
will work the ground for food in order to live. It will be
painful and difficult, as your efforts will produce both
eatable and non-eatable results. You will eat cursed
produce from the ground, and you will return to the
ground*
(Davidson, 2003).

Prior to sin, it is neither stated nor implied that food is necessary to sustain life (Genesis 1:29; 2:9). Prior to sin, the occurrence of the Hebrew term (makal, i.e., food) in Genesis means the fruit or herb is eatable. Clearly, eating was for enjoyment and pleasure. This is why the serpent's lure was so appealing to the woman. As the serpent would have it, the "forbidden" fruit was not merely for enjoyment and pleasure. The forbidden fruit offered exceptional capabilities (Genesis 3:5). Notice what the woman perceives when she "locks-in" on the forbidden fruit. She saw that the forbidden fruit was, "… good for food, and that it was a delight to the eyes, and that the tree was desirable to make one wise, she took from its fruit and ate…" (Genesis 3:6, NASB). If we hold that eating was necessary to sustain life before sin, then it is an admission that the first man and woman lived under the authority of death. While the potential for sin was represented in man's environment (Genesis 2:17, Genesis 3:1, Romans 5:12), the Biblical fact is that man did not live under the authority of death until after sin.

Emphatically, it appears that only one tree was designated as the source of sustenance. This was the life sustaining tree (Genesis 3:24). Theologians reason that man was expelled from the garden, and the tree of life was guarded. This prevented man from eating from the tree of life. Apparently, the tree could sustain their lives even under the conditions of sin. However, this does not mean that they had to eat from the tree of life to live before the first sin.

Because of the curses related to Adam (Genesis 3:17-19), we need food to sustain our lives, but food is also a contributor to the dying process. I do not mean only food with destructive content (e.g., processes, chemicals, various fats, cholesterol, etc.). Since the ground is cursed, food is cursed. Therefore, food in general contributes to the dying process. Given man's conduct, God cursed what was designed as a pleasure (i.e., Genesis 1:29, 2:9) and changed it to a source of the dying process. It is amazing. Eating is a topic or cause in the original prohibition (Genesis 2:17), original sin (Genesis 3:6), and original curses (Genesis 3:17-19).

Once the believer understands the Biblical insights as stated above, it adds a new and different perspective to fasting.

By Bread Alone

Most of the illustrations of fasting occur in the Old Testament (1 Kings 19:8; Deuteronomy 9:9-18; Exodus 34:28; Joel 2:12; I Samuel 14:24; 2 Chronicles 20:3; 34:28; Ezra 10:6; Esther 4:16). Fasting is also found in the New Testament (Matthew 17:21; Mark 9:29; Acts 10:30; 1 Corinthians 7:5).

However, Jesus must be the center focus, particularly His instruction about fasting. It is noteworthy that when Jesus is going to launch into His earthly ministry it begins with an extended period of fasting. This is an extended fast because Biblically only two other people fasted similarly. The majority of fasts found in the Bible are seven days or less. Nevertheless, there are some noteworthy facts about the fast, which Jesus practiced.

It is a progressive fast. It is more of the Mosaic type fast where Jesus is about to launch into a new phase in His life. This is similar to Moses when God gave him the Law. Jesus' fast is for both physical and spiritual purposes. Notice that afterward Jesus is hungry, and Satan is on the scene as he was in the Garden of Eden (Matthew 4:2). Imagine! Jesus' first recorded temptation is to turn stones into bread. How ironic! The first man, Adam succumbed to eating and Satan tries the same ploy with Jesus. No wonder Paul states, "...for we are not ignorant of his devices" (2 Corinthians 2:11, NASB). Nevertheless, Jesus' reply to Satan's temptation is priceless for us today:

But he answered and said, It is written, Man shall not live by bread alone, but by every word that proceedeth out of the mouth of God
(Matthew 4:4, KJV).

When Jesus said, "...Man shall not live by bread alone." What does He mean by "live"? Generically, one could conclude that He means spiritually or eternally. However, in the context of the question and His condition of hunger, Jesus meant physically. Physically, man does not live by bread alone. Obviously, he also lives by periods of abstaining from food. Jesus' fast was not only concerning His spiritual preparation. Ministry requires thorough preparation spiritually, physically, psychologically, and socially. Jesus knew the facts about food consumption.

While we must eat, eating also reduces life expectancy if it is not controlled. There are numerous spiritual advantages fasting affords. Jesus also teaches us by his example to control food consumption by fasting for our physical well-being. Jesus said, "Man shall not live by bread alone…" He refused to turn the stone to bread, and He certainly did not eat. What a striking image for us today.

PART II
Beyond Fasting

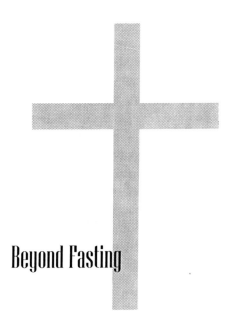

Beyond Fasting

God's Word Teaches Content and Portion

Most believers do not realize that there are dietary guidelines provided in the Bible. Based on the effect of sin, man moved from being an eater for enjoyment, to eating for survival. Sin caused him to degenerate from plant or fruit consumption to consuming animal life. This major change takes place after the flood (Genesis 9:2-5; Leviticus 11; Deuteronomy 14). Notice that the basic framework for eating animals is that they could not be carnivorous animals. Animals and insects of prey or scavengers were to be avoided. The instructions clearly preferred animals who survived on plant-life. Animal consumption was clearly an alternative for survival, and not the preferable design to sustain man.

Keep in mind, animals where not originally designed to be consumed. Apparently, due to the damage upon the ecosystem of the earth after the flood, man is instructed to eat animals or insects to augment his dietary needs. While the new animal diet supplements the original plant-based diet, it is not coincidental that man's life expectancy decreases dramatically after the flood.

The Bible's view of an uncontrolled appetite is clear. The Bible casts gluttony along with alcoholism or drunkenness (Deuteronomy 21:20, Proverbs 23:21). Many of us are guilty when it comes to gluttony. Given the typical person in our culture, we are consumed with eating. Think about it. We eat on every occasion, and everywhere we go. We are the gluttony generation. We eat at ball games, movies, parks, work, play, and church. Recall, Jesus was accused of being an alcoholic and gluttonous (Matthew 11:19, Luke 7:34). The Greek term "phagos" was used to characterize and label Jesus as a man who over indulged himself eating. Today, many of us are familiar with this term in a different context, but with the same demeaning impact. The English cognate, fagot is the derogatory slur used to berate a homosexual. The term is an obvious reference to the person who indulges beyond the gender limit, sexually. However, the sting of being called a glutton in Jesus' day was exponentially worse in comparison.

As a Matter of Course, Often Jesus Did Not Eat

It was not only a lie to call Jesus a glutton, it was utterly preposterous. While Jesus certainly consumed food, it was not unusual for Him to go days without eating. These were not periods when He was fasting. These were periods when he was so engaged in ministry, food did not dominate his attention. Moreover, the evidence suggests that his disciples also practiced sheer abstinence from food. There are several experiences in His life where this truth is obvious.

Jesus' encounter with the woman at the well concluded with his disciples offering Jesus something to eat. Jesus responded, "I have food to eat that you do not know about." We may assume that Jesus is talking about being strengthened spiritually, and who is to argue such a conclusion. However, it does not exclude the fact that it was also nourishing His physical body. The context of the food offered is physical food for physical strength. No doubt, His reply is in reference to the physical nourishment the food offers (John 4:31-33). Therefore, His spiritual nourishment was also empowering His physical body. They did not realize that the Spirit nourishes the spiritual and physical.

There were several occasions when Jesus ministered to thousands of people. There was one occasion when the disciples were hungry, and they asked Jesus to send the crowd away to lodge and eat. Clearly, the people had not eaten. It seems to indicate that the disciples where really the ones who desired to eat. So, Jesus told His disciples to feed the crowd. They were dumb founded because they only had enough food for themselves. Subsequently, Jesus feeds the people with five loaves and two fish (Matthew 14:9, Luke 9:12-17). However, as in the encounter with the woman at the well, thousands had not eaten for days without a complaint.

Again, Jesus ministers to thousands of people (Matthew 15:32-36). They have been with Him three days, and they had not eaten. This time He has to inform his disciples they cannot send the people away without eating. Obviously, the disciples have matured to a point where going without food as a matter of course is the norm. His circle of disciples plus thousands who have gone without food represents a remarkable virtue we often miss as believers.

It was not news for persons involved in the Christ-based Weight Management program when an astonishing scientific finding was reported in the Dallas Morning News, July 26 2004. The article revealed the following:

> *In the fractious field of aging research, the benefit of reducing calories is one of the few areas of agreement. This means much more than just skipping dessert. It's taking relatively severe steps, such as slashing calories by as much as two-thirds or eating only every other day, which increases life span, studies suggest.*

Whether or not the scientific community ever comes to a final determination, numerous participants have noticed major physical and bodily improvements (e.g., skin tone, digestive regularity, improved test results, etc.). These all improve participant's physical quality of life. No scientist knows human anatomy like Jesus. Jesus did not allow food to dominate His life, and the same can be said for His followers.

All Things Are Clean

After making such a profound finding, it is profitable to discuss what Paul states about food offered to idols in his letters to the Roman and Corinthian churches:

Do not tear down the work of God for the sake of food.
All things indeed are clean, but they are evil for the man
who eats and gives offense. It is good not to eat meat or
to drink wine, or to do anything by which your brother
stumbles
(Romans 14:20-21)

As concerning therefore the eating of those things that
are offered in sacrifice unto idols, we know that an idol
is nothing in the world, and that there is none other God
but one. For though there be that are called gods,
whether in heaven or in earth, (as there be gods many,
and lords many,) But to us there is but one God, the
Father, of whom are all things, and we in him; and one
Lord Jesus Christ, by whom are all things, and we by
him. Howbeit there is not in every man that knowledge:
for some with conscience of the idol unto this hour eat it
as a thing offered unto an idol; and their conscience
being weak is defiled. But meat commendeth us not to
God: for neither, if we eat, are we the better; neither, if
we eat not, are we the worse
(I Corinthians 8:4-8, KJV)

We should not confuse Paul's statements concerning food offered to idols with the origin of food as sustenance. The issue is the spiritual implications of eating meat offered to idols. Paul explains that all things are clean. Again, in the context of Paul's statements, he means the meat is not somehow "extraordinarily" cursed because it is offered to idols. He affirms this in his letter to Corinthians where he explains, "an idol is nothing in the world, and there is none other God but one." Therefore, Paul's instructions do not discuss the basic truth about food in general.

Paul's instructions to Timothy are similarly based on the same issue, where meat was offered to idols. There were persons who taught believers to abstain from this "meat" offered to idols.

Now the Spirit speaketh expressly, that in the latter
times some shall depart from the faith, giving heed to
seducing spirits, and doctrines of devils; speaking lies in
hypocrisy; having their conscience seared with a hot

iron; Forbidding to marry, and commanding to <u>abstain</u>
<u>from meats</u>, which God hath created to be received with
thanksgiving of them which believe and know the truth
(I Timothy 4:1-3)

Again, the clause, "abstaining from meats" has nothing to do with fasting. Paul adds an interesting insight about physical nourishment. He states,

For every creature of God is good, and nothing to be
refused, if it be received with thanksgiving: For it is
sanctified by the word of God and prayer. If thou put
the brethren in remembrance of these things, thou shalt
be a good minister of Jesus Christ, <u>nourished up in the</u>
<u>words of faith and of good doctrine</u>, whereunto thou
hast attained
(I. Timothy 4:4-6, KJV)

Believers must exercise caution when viewing Paul's words that every creature of God is good, and that food is sanctified by the Word of God and prayer. Paul is not mincing words. He means it is good. It is set apart for eating, and there are no spiritual or sin implications involved with eating the food. However, note the comparison between food's nourishment for the body, and the words of faith for the body. The body receives nutritional strength by words of faith. Obedience to God's Word relative to our body wellness is much more profitable than physical efforts (e.g., exercise, right foods, examinations, etc.). This is further affirmed by Paul when he states,

But refuse profane and old wives' fables, and exercise
thyself rather unto godliness. For bodily exercise
profiteth little: but godliness is profitable unto all
things, having promise of the life that now is, and of that
which is to come
(I Timothy 4:7-8, KJV)

Compared to principles of faith related to our bodies, physical exercise does not compare favorably. He states, "godliness is profitable unto <u>all things</u>." Paul is speaking of both the physical body and spiritual life. Both the physical life and spiritual life is further indicated when he says, "for the life that now <u>is</u>, and of that which is <u>to come</u>."

However, returning to I Corinthian 6:12-13, we can determine how Paul views food related to the topic in this book. He provides excellent insight into both the cursed characteristics of food and the digestive system. They are both the result of sin, and shall be destroyed. That is, they will not be a part of our glorified bodies. As with Jesus after the resurrection, we can eat food, but there is no digestive process. What happens to the food is a mystery (Luke 24:42; John 21:13).

Exercise and proper diet have obvious benefit. However, the point is clear, the Word of God is more important to bodily wellness than exercise or other similar activities. Issues such as lifestyle and food abstinence or fasting lead the way concerning God's Word related to physical wellness.

PART III

Empowerment for a Lifetime

The Spiritual Aspect of Consumption Control

Dieting has become a multi-billion dollar industry. Schemes, tricks, scams, and shams are quick methods of earning money from those who desire to control eating. Interestingly, we pray about most issues concerning our health. How often does a person pray and fast for consumption control? Have you ever thought about fasting for bodily health? What a novel idea! Consumption control is directly related to weight control, and weight control to bodily health. Paul calls the body, the temple of the Holy Spirit (I Corinthians 6:19-20). He made this statement concerning the effect of sin upon the body. However, the point is clear. The body is used to glorify God, and physical health relates directly to our ability to perform the Great Commission (Matthew 28:18-20).

Fasting, an Unpopular Necessity

Many of the most prestigious mainline denominations do little to support fasting. There are those who hold a view that fasting is not a principle to exercise today. There are those who believe it is a principle exercised under the Law. Admittedly, fasting is not a major theme in the doctrinal books of the New Testament (Romans, Corinthians, Colossians, etc.). Fasting is a factor when the Church is launched (Acts 10:30, Acts 14:23, Acts 27:33). Paul further indicates that it is a part of the believer's personal strength discipline (I Corinthian 7:5). It is not clear why it is not mentioned more significantly in the apostolic writings (e.g., Paul, Peter, John, etc.). Nevertheless, Jesus intended for fasting to be a discipline in the believer's life. When asked why His disciples did not fast, Jesus responded as follows:

> *You cannot make the attendants of the bridegroom fast*
> *while the bridegroom is with them, can you? "But the*
> *days will come; and when the bridegroom is taken away*
> *from them, then they will fast in those days"*
> *(Luke 5:34-35; see also*
> *Matthew 9:14; Mark 2:18)*

A person may believe that "those days" means the days between Jesus' death and resurrection. However, this view is defeated by fasting and exhortations to fast, which occurred after Jesus resurrection (Acts 14:23; Acts 27:33, I Corinthians 7:5). Therefore, fasting is relevant for the current Church Age, or Age of Grace. Furthermore, Jesus seems to indicate a new or expanded purpose for fasting. After indicating that believers are to fast after he departs, Jesus adds,

> *And he spake also a parable unto them; No man putteth*
> *a piece of a new garment upon an old; if otherwise, then*
> *both the new maketh a rent, and the piece that was taken*
> *out of the new agreeth not with the old. And no man*
> *putteth new wine into old bottles; else the new wine will*
> *burst the bottles, and be spilled, and the bottles shall*
> *perish. But new wine must be put into new bottles; and*
> *both are preserved*
> *(Luke 5:36-38 KJV)*

When viewing the other Gospels on the same topic (Matt 9:14, Mark 2:18), it appears that this parable is a continuation of Jesus' point about fasting. Contextually, this new and expanded purpose for fasting is progressive and visionary. This is in contrast to the more reflective, remorseful, or repentant modes under the Law. This new and progressive fasting is affirmed by Jesus' disclosure concerning a boy possessed by demons. The disciples were unsuccessful when they attempted to heal the boy. They asked Jesus why they could not cure the boy. Jesus replied, "But this kind does not go out except by prayer and fasting" (Matthew 17:21). Did Jesus mean that once they saw the boy they needed to begin praying and fasting? No! Obviously, Jesus meant that the level of ministry involving demons required a discipline or practice of prayer and fasting. This would provide both the spiritual and physical strength needed to exorcise the demon when needed. The type of fasting Jesus introduces is ministry related fasting. Fasting when coupled with prayer provides strength for ministry.

The point here is that fasting is an overlooked necessity for the believer's life. However, our love for food consumption is so pervasive, we do not like anything limiting our food intake or content. Therefore, fasting is one of the least likely Christian necessities a believer will practice.

Building the Fast Threshold

Returning to Jesus' wilderness experience, please note that he was hungry after the fast (Matthew 4:2). This sounds incredulous, but persons who fast regularly experience it. The more often a person fasts, the person builds a "fasting threshold." That is, the body begins to accommodate the fast. Since the hunger most of us encounter is "psycho addictive," it is overcome with practice. This means that most of our responses to fasting are going to be mental. Headaches, weakness, nervousness and similar manifestations are all mental. Believers must understand that fasting is not dieting. Fasting has spiritual implications. The more a person fasts, the body begins to adjust and allow the person to fast without withdrawal manifestations such as headaches, weakness, hunger pains, etc. It is important to discuss any weight management program with your physician.

Since obesity significantly reduces life expectancy, people are opting for gastro-intestinal surgery, or stomach stapling as a last chance. The net effect of these drastic procedures is that they dramatically reduce food intake. The person simply does not have the capacity to eat large volumes of food. This demonstrates how drastic dieting has to be in order to lose significant amounts of weight. This is why most people are not successful.

However, fasting can have the same result as these major surgeries. After an extended fast of three days or more, it is not unusual that the stomach has already tightened. The person cannot eat as usual. This is an important consumption reduction factor. In addition, fasting combines one of the most powerful elements of the mind and soul to physical wellness. Faith!

A person's personal faith is extremely powerful. Where a person may lack the personal will to diet, the answer may be found in the Christ-based fast. One's "belief" conviction is so deep, it may be the decisive success factor. Upon recognizing that fasting is a central part of the believer's life, there will be persons who will succeed where they could not previously. This further emphasizes the importance of believing God's Word concerning the body. It is the temple of the Holy Spirit.

Also, it is important that fasting be combined with morning prayer, a singular focus, and full schedule. As alluded to above, the Christ-based fast is not monk-like. The person maintains a typical schedule to the degree possible.

Establishing a Fast Pattern

Recall the experience where the young lad was possessed by a demon, and the disciples could not heal him. When asked why they were not successful, Jesus explained the need for prayer and fasting. As stated above, he meant a practice of prayer and fasting. People who have an established prayer life typically have a time and place for prayer. Believers should also establish a fast schedule. While this may sound scripted or mechanical, the term disciple has as its origin, in the word "discipline." If a person is fasting for bodily wellness, the following is recommended:

- Begin by attempting to fast for seven days. Set your goal for seven days, and pray for success. If this is not possible, fast as many days as possible. The person can eat one meal, and continue fasting. Some people use the 3+3+1 method. They fast three days and eat one meal. Fast another three days, and eat a meal. And then fast one day and eat a meal. People who are extremely weight challenged should employ a forty day fast. The value to the person's life expectancy and quality of life is well worth an extended fast. <u>Again, a physician must be consulted before embarking on any weight management program.</u>

▪ Once you resume eating, you will become full rather quickly. You should stop eating.

▪ Remember, the battle is going to be mental. It is important to drink fluids such as 100% fruit juices (e.g., Apple, Orange, Grape, etc.) and water. Dehydration is much more an issue than starvation. As the CDC statistics show, there are not too many people who have to worry about starvation in our culture. Nevertheless, stock up with fruit juices and water. A complete list of nutrients and other considerations are in the Program Tools section.

▪ When hunger rises, respond with the words, "Man does not live by bread alone, but every word that proceeds from the mouth of God;" or respond with whatever techniques and spiritual responses a believer prefers.

▪ Once the believer completes the first full week, resume with a weekly fast schedule. Use discretion to determine the span of days that work for you (e.g., 1 day, 2 day). The more extensive your regular fast period (e.g., 3 days), the more results you will experience.

▪ While you can begin the fast anytime, it is best to begin the fast at the beginning of the week. Most people on the program begin their fast with the last meal on Sunday (i.e., dinner), and conclude it with dinner on Tuesday. Again, if beginning Sunday does not fit, do what is suitable.

If a believer maintains the schedule, it will become easier and easier. Notice what is happening physically when you maintain this schedule. The believer is dramatically reducing calories by as much as 28%.

So, if a believer is consuming about 2000 calories a day, this amounts to 14,000 calories a week. Once a believer begins fasting, this is cut to 10,000 calories per week. Persons who fast for forty days reduce the annual caloric intake by as much as 80,000 calories or 10% in a little over a month. If the believer resumes eating after the fast with regular dieting, this is very dramatic compared to dieting alone. Additionally, employing a spiritual principle offers a powerful dimension otherwise unavailable. As the believer builds the fasting threshold, it is not unusual to fast three days or more regularly.

Within one week, the believer will notice some amazing results. Yes, there will be water weight reduction, but more specifically the digestive system is cleared of gases and other toxins from the food. Since weight loss is slow, it is very valuable to focus on the other more immediate advantages. There is also a spiritual component where one is given a greater sense of spiritual fullness.

Forty Day Period and Personal Resolve

No one should expect dramatic weight loss results for at least forty days. I speak about the forty-day period at great length in the Process of Being Made Whole. Typically, when the believer stays on course for forty or more days, it is evidence of faith and resolve. A believer's mind must be convinced that fasting will be done for the remainder of one's life. It is not a temporary principle and practice. Most people did not gain the excess weight in a forty-day period, and it will not be removed in a forty-day period. Forty days simply establishes in the spirit realm that the believer is faithful, and the believer is determined to improve one's physical wellness.

"eXaltorcise" Insights

As opposed to exercise, persons in the Christ-based Weight Management program adopted the term "eXaltorcise" (i.e., exalt–or–cise). This term has a Biblical basis. First, the Greek letter X is the first letter in the word Christ. X has the phonetic "key" sound. We use the English phonetic "ex" sound such as exalt. Exalt means to lift or raise an object. Specifically, the person in the program exalts Jesus Christ through the physical activity. The stem of the word (i.e., "orcise") is a truncated form of exorcise (i.e., eliminate, or expel). There is a lot of misinformation about how much "eXaltorcise" is required in order for a person to control one's weight. We need to be frankly honest. Given the typical person who does not eXaltorcise, it is going to take a major effort. Obviously, persons with a regular eXaltorcise routine may only need to modify one's current program. Typically, weight loss requires about forty minutes of eXaltorcise. Forty minutes may sound like a lot of time each day. However, the typical person watches T.V. far more than forty minutes per day. Considering the importance and value concerned with personal wellness, there should be substantial motivation for an eXaltorcise program. Some believers eXaltorcise two or more times a day for twenty minutes.

EXaltorcise requires an elevated heart rate. So, walking while helpful may not contribute to weight loss. Therefore, the person has to walk briskly to get the advantage of burning calories.

Unfortunately, eXaltorcise can be difficult for persons who are extremely weight challenged. However, eXaltorcise includes a focus on God's healing hand as he inhabits our eXaltorcise period (Psalms 42:11, 43:5, 63:5). Remember, it is God's will and design that we take care of our bodily temples. Nevertheless, most eXaltorcise routines (e.g., walking, jogging, biking, etc.) can cause structural or joint pain. Persons should use creativity to the degree possible. There are many vehicles available for eXaltorcise (treadmills, stair-steppers, cross-trainers, etc.). One of the best eXaltorcise vehicles for persons with excessive weight is the recumbent bike. The recumbent bike allows a person to sit with back support for the mass of weight on the posterior. Some recumbent bikes also have vertical eXaltorcise handles, which operate to invigorate the upper body. While eXaltorcise equipment can be expensive, recumbent bikes are offered as low as $100.00 at Wal Mart. Remember, eXaltorcise equipment can be deducted from taxes as a medical expense. A physician must recommend the equipment for health. See your physician and tax consultant for more information.

Locate the bike or other equipment in an area where you can watch television or listen to other multimedia programming. Music should have a strong Christian message. Remember, the eXaltorcise is primary, and any multimedia enhancement is secondary. It is not unusual to see people exercising with books and newspapers barely incurring a sweat. While most physical activity or typical exercise is helpful, it offers little or no value toward weight loss. The bottom line is to find a regular eXaltorcise routine.

An added incentive for eXaltorcise is the immediate impact it can have on hypertension. I stumbled upon this when I happened to take a blood pressure reading following a workout. I discovered that my blood pressure was well below my baseline reading. Dr. Kenneth Cooper an expert on hypertension affirms what I discovered. He has found that when a person exercises for an extended period (e.g., 35 to 40 minutes), one can experience a decrease in blood pressure[2]. Again, this is for persons who can sustain an aerobic workout for several minutes. When this is apparent, a person may be able to control hypertension with aerobic eXaltorcise as opposed to medicinal therapy. Persons desiring to control hypertension with aerobic eXaltorcise must consult with a physician. Remember, believers should "eXaltorcise" and not just exercise. Finally, regardless of the intensity of your "eXaltorcise" program, it must be combined with significant caloric reduction or weight loss results will be negligible.

Myths, Concerns, and Observations

A small or slim body means good shape: First, a brief explanation of the term "good shape" is required. Often the term means the person is not overweight, and has an appearance of physical wellness. Simply because someone has a small frame does not mean that he or she is in good shape. Persons need a regular physician's evaluation to determine levels of cholesterol, blood sugar, and other indicators.

A muscular frame means good shape: There are persons who prefer isometric (i.e., resistance training), as opposed to aerobic (i.e., cardio vascular) exercise. A muscular frame does not mean a person is in good shape. Again, persons need a physician's evaluation. Persons particularly prefer isometric activities because it adds definition to the body. Persons who suffer with hypertension must be cautious about isometric activities. Cooper[3] warns that weight-training activities can promote hypertension. I noticed a middle-aged woman who often participated in isometric activities. She exercised daily with isometric equipment. I asked her if she had difficulties with hypertension. She informed me that she was recently diagnosed. I informed her about Dr. Cooper's findings. She had no idea that weight training could contribute to hypertension. Again, persons who participate in any of these activities should consult a physician.

I personally use a 2 to 1 approach. Beginning with cardio vascular

---

[2] Cooper, Overcoming Hypertension, 183
[3] Ibid, 181

activities, I participate in cardio vascular activities two times more than resistance training (i.e., isometric, weight training. etc.). Consult with your physician concerning an approach acceptable for you.

A person in good shape cannot have a stroke or heart attack: No one regardless of physical conditioning can assume such a guarantee. The medical community speaks in terms of risk factors. Obesity and related problems increase the risk of a major stroke, heart attack, and related illnesses. Therefore, everyone has some degree of risk.

Protein based diet: Simply because a program contributes to weight loss does not mean it improves the overall health profile. There is a lot of controversy concerning the Atkins diet. The Atkins diet is referred to as a high protein diet. Since animal meat provides protein, the focus is to trade-off carbohydrates for protein. While it has been found to be successful for some people to help them lose weight, the high fat content in animal meat must be a major concern. Again, losing weight is not the only purpose for weight management. The purpose is to improve a person's health profile including weight, and related health factors (e.g., brain, heart, lungs, etc.). The Bible clearly does not support eating high animal meat content as our daily staple. Apparently, red meat was a delicacy reserved for special days (1Samuel 28:24, Proverbs 15:17, Matthew 22:4, Luke 15: 23, 27).

Dieting vs. Fasting: Some people will find fasting more hassle free than dieting. Dieting requires constant concern with caloric intake. The dieter must carefully choose what will be consumed. There are no such issues with the person who is fasting. Other than water and juices, which are typically low in calories compared to typical food consumption, there is little concern about calories. Both are similar concerning enticements, and the temptation to eat. However, there is also no concern about over-eating on a given day for the person who fasts. If a person is employing the Christ-based fast, over eating is impossible during the fast. Any one who diets regularly knows over-eating is a constant concern for the dieter.

When the weight goal is reached, eXaltorcise is not necessary: EXaltorcise is necessary even when a person reaches her/his target weight. Among other advantages, eXaltorcise speeds the flow of the blood stream, which operates like a high-speed rinse of blood passageways. This helps to remove plaque type particles, which cause major health events such as a heart attack or stroke. These plaque materials are dispensed through the body's removal system (e.g., sweat glands, bowels, etc.). Regardless of the weight status, eXaltorcise is a positive physical and spiritual health factor. <u>As stated before, persons considering an exercise program must consult with a physician.</u>

PROGRAM
TOOLS

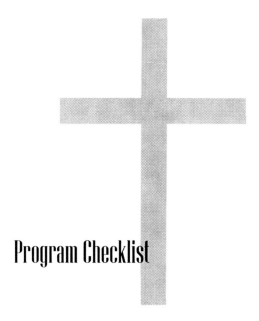

Program Checklist

- ☐ Complete the Process of Being Made Whole including all the questions.
- ☐ Completely read Christ-based Weight Management.
- ☐ Read the Covenant, and Program Notes and Handouts section of the CBWM book.
- ☐ Take your initial weight before starting the Seven Days of Heaven fast. Mark this weight on your covenant (page 1 of 5).
- ☐ The Seven Days of Heaven fast begins at 11:59:59 p.m. Sunday (3+3+1 fast).
- ☐ The first period of the fast is concluded at 4:00 p.m. Wednesday.
- ☐ The second fast period begins at 11:59:59 pm Wednesday night.
- ☐ The second fast period is concluded at 4:00 p.m. Saturday.
- ☐ The final day of fasting begins at 11:59:59 Saturday night.
- ☐ The Seven Days of Heaven are concluded at 4:00 p.m. on Sunday.
- ☐ Weigh yourself at the end of the fast period. Mark this on your covenant (page 1 of 5).

☐ Again, read the Covenant, and Program Notes and Handouts, Understanding the Program Design (i.e., page 1 of 5 on your covenant).

☐ Decide, which level of program you will begin and initial, sign, and date the covenant with witnesses. Begin the fast period you selected when you have completed the Seven Days of Heaven.

☐ Each week answer 50 questions in your CBWM Counseling guide. You MUST finish 50 per week. DO NOT complete more than 50 per week.

☐ Submit the questions via the internet to CBWMprogram@aol.com each week.

☐ DAILY, refer to the 7 Powerful Christ-based Truths about Gluttony and Deliverance. The can be found on the Christ-based Counseling web site at Christbasedcounseling.org.

☐ Conduct your 45-day weigh-in. Mark this weight on your covenant (page 1 of 5).

☐ Weigh yourself according to the schedule as stated in the Covenant, and Program Notes and Handouts.

☐ If you have questions send them to CBWMprogram@aol.com

NOTE: It is strongly recommended that you consult a physician before beginning any weight management program

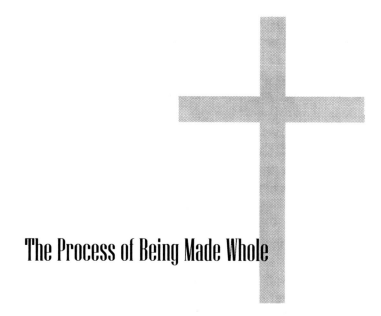

The Process of Being Made Whole

The core of Christ-based Counseling (CBC) is the Process of Being Made Whole. This Process includes six constituents and strategic prayer for forty-five days. Regardless of the issue, it is important for the counselee to understand these factors.

The Counselee Must Be Born-Again (John 3:3-8): The foundation of Christ-based Counseling's effectiveness is in the faith dimension. Therefore, only persons who are believers can avail themselves to the therapeutic or healing process in Christ-based Counseling. Persons who do not know the Lord, but desire CBC must be evangelized first. Nevertheless, Jesus' discussion with Nicodemus in the referenced text makes the point clear. The counselee must be born again.

The Counselee Must Be Presented Balanced Biblical Insights (Matt. 4:5-7): God's Word, rightly divided is the therapy for right thinking. However as shown in the referenced text, God's Word must be balanced, and not some half-concocted, or perverted presentation of God's Word. This can be seen in the Devil's inappropriate use of Psalms 91. Christ-based Counseling relies on the appropriate use of God's Word, and understands the overarching principles of God's

Word.

The Counselee Must Possess the Degree of Faith Needed (Mark 4:24): Beyond possessing faith unto salvation, counselees must believe that God will intervene in their personal circumstances. The referenced verse is preceded by verses 13-20 where Jesus explains the different types of hearers of God's Word: Wayside, Stony, Thorns & Thistles, and Good Ground. Each of these persons represents how "hearers" embrace God's Word. Regardless of the circumstances, Good Ground hearers <u>believe</u>. They believe that God "is" operating in their personal situation.

The Counselee Must Be Committed (Luke 21:1-4): Counselees must be thoroughly invested in the Process. The woman in the example gave "all" that she had. What a difference she represents compared to the typical person in our culture. Often people do not desire to make the investment of time and personal sacrifice. This Process requires complete commitment by the counselee as the woman shown in the referenced text.

The Counselee Must Do The Practical (Mark 8:1-3): Depending on the issue, counselees must do the practical or physical things. As shown in the referenced text, Jesus recognizes the need to feed the multitude, or they would faint. The practical matters must be satisfied, and these are usually understood. As an example, a person seeking a job must seek employment opportunities, and submit applications where applicable.

The Counselee Must Stay In The Process (John 15:3-9): Persons who encounter any issue must be willing to invest time in counseling, prayer, study, and application of God's Word. It is popular to look for the immediate answer and quick solution. However, the essence of a problem is that the answer may not result in an immediate resolution. Therefore, counselees must stay in the counseling process as scheduled. Also, they must be engaged in the greater fellowship of believers, and on-going development in Christ.

Forty-Five Days of Prayer

Important to the counseling process is the additional therapeutic dimension of strategic prayer. As opposed to generalized prayer, the term strategic is used to denote the specific focus of prayer. Remember, Christ-based Counseling works with both dimensions (i.e., the natural and spiritual). The Lord has empowered believers to impact the spiritual dimension.

Why Forty-five Days? As mentioned in the sixth constituent of the Process of Being Made Whole, issues faced by most counselees represent problems that will not be resolved in a short timeframe. Additionally, many believers do not have a daily and concentrated prayer regimen.

Most important life changes require a transition, which usually involves the combination of an established timeframe and a different behavioral pattern, focus, or practice.

Biblically, the number forty is used so often it is more than a mere coincident. Other significant numbers, which most of us hear about are three and seven. There are others not mentioned as significantly.

One must be cautious about the use of numbers. There is always the danger that one may be overcome by superstition and mysticism involving numbers. Praying for forty-five days has nothing to do with any kind of superstition.

Biblically, [after sin] it appears that it requires a timeframe of about forty earth days or years for the operation of angels to complete an assignment. The term, "earth days" are used for our (i.e., human) benefit. Angels are the purveyors of God's will. That is, they are the workers at God's command who cause results in the material universe. God uses the angels to create, change, or allow our circumstances. They work in the angelic dimension, but their results are manifested in the physical dimension. Clearly, God has connected our prayers to their operation. There are more than 250 references to angels in the Bible.

Since angels are not limited by time or space, they merely refer to days for our benefit (e.g., Dan. 10:13). Therefore, the events in Scripture involving "forty" often refer to the completion of a phase, process, or administration. If this is true, the principle should be witnessed at least three times in Scripture (Deuteronomy 17:6; Matthew 18:16). Examples are provided as follows:

Genesis 7:12: It rained forty days and forty nights (i.e. the Flood) before the renewal of the earth.

Numbers 13:25: Moses commissioned spies to assess the land for forty days. They returned before making their final decision concerning the Promised Land. When they were found to be unfaithful, they wandered for forty years.

Deuteronomy 10:10: Both times the tablets of the Ten

Commandments required forty days to complete before being presented to the Hebrews.

I Kings 19:5-8: Prompted by two angels to eat, afterwards, Elijah fasts for forty days and nights before journeying to Mt. Horeb. There, he received transition instructions.

Ezekiel 4:6: God instructed the prophet to lie on his side for forty days as an object lesson to Judah representing the years of Judah's iniquity.

Daniel 10:13, 20: Bewildered about a vision, Daniel prays for understanding. The angel reveals that it took him twenty-one days to arrive, but the angel's mission was not concluded. He had to return and continue his battle with the prince of Persia--at least another 21 days.

Jonah 3:4: The prophet warned Nineveh that it had forty days before being overthrown. They repented and averted their doom.

The Old Testament is where the precedent is found for the significance of a timeframe covering at least forty days. More importantly, there are two extraordinary events in the life of Jesus involving forty-day periods. **First**, the gospels (Matthew 4:2; Mark 1:3; Luke 4:2) record Jesus' wilderness journey before initiating His earthly ministry. This period launching His earthly ministry was forty days and forty nights. Angels were on the scene ministering to Him (Matt. 4:11; Mark 1:13). **Secondly**, as an irrefutable demonstration of His resurrection, Jesus appeared and ministered for a period of forty days (Acts 1:3). Again, angels were on the scene as He departed earth (Acts 1:10-11).

It is noteworthy here that one of the important characteristics Jesus taught about prayer was persistency (Luke 11:5-8; Luke 18:1-8). Luke 18:1 provides the specific purpose for the instructions on prayer. Pointedly, He instructed that we must not <u>loose heart</u> (KJV) or <u>give up</u> (NIV). The Apostle Paul used terms such as "pray without ceasing" and "always praying" (Eph. 6:18; Col. 1:3; I Th. 5:17).

Recall the case where a boy was psychotic (Matt. 17:14-21), and the disciples could not cure him. Jesus rebuked the demon in the boy, and he was cured. The disciples wanted to know why they could not cure the boy. Jesus identified the problem: Their lack of faith demonstrated by the absence of prayer and fasting. Persistency in prayer is the evidence of faithfulness. Therefore, Jesus did not mean they did not pray at the moment of need. He meant, "This could only be done by persons with a discipline of prayer and fasting." The most challenging issues in life require a process of faith demonstrated by persistent prayer disciplines (i.e., prayer and fasting). Disciples/persons with these virtues need only to strategically focus on a specific need. Like Jesus, their angels are "on-the-ready" awaiting marching orders from the Lord (Matt. 18:10; 26:51-53). **NOTE:** Believers must not worship, or pray to angels.

Clearly, Jesus knew the reality of what happens in the angelic dimension when believers pray. The angels are on the move, but they are opposed. God has connected their success to our faith or persistence. Jesus says, "don't loose heart." We must keep praying on a specific issue.

Finally, Ephesians 6:10-20 discusses the opposition to believers' walk in Christ. Paul makes it clear that the overwhelming objective must be to defeat demonic operations in the angelic dimension. Once this is accomplished, the way is cleared for "results" in the physical or material dimension. Please notice that the weaponry is spiritual. The Christ-based Counseling focus is verses 16-18. These verses highlight faith, the Spirit or Word of God, and prayer as the primary weapons. Paul adds, "… and watching with all perseverance …" No doubt, God can resolve a matter in a day. However, the Biblical evidence is convincing that a process is required for matters requiring spiritual intervention.

Finally, the term, "forty years" is also noteworthy. "Forty-years" is used more often than "forty-days." Consider that with God and the angels, there is no difference between forty-days, and forty-years (Psalms 90:4; 2 Peter 3:8). When believers pray in a range of forty days--in God's will, they will see a discernable change. Remember, this affirms a process or practice in the angelic dimension. The issue may not be resolved, but there will be change. In addition, a person will be closer to the Lord's answer. Obviously, some matters of prayer will be with us a lifetime. Others are not long at all.

Test it! If you have an issue, follow the six-steps, and pray forty-five days. See if there is an affirmative "change." Remember, the number, "forty" is not magical. One is to keep praying until the mission is complete.

Who is the origin of the additional five days? As Paul would say, "this is not the Lord's command, but mine and I believe it is worthy. An additional five days cannot hurt." sbd

College of Professional Christian Studies (Global)
Departments of Biblical Studies and Christ-based Counseling

COURSE: Process of Being Made Whole (6 constituents and 45 days of prayer)

Practicum Requirement:

Course Literature: CBC Study and Bible

Pre-requisites (if any):

Understanding the Course Design:

   Students use the literature to respond to questions. Questions are in chronological order throughout the course. Questions preceded with bracket statements require Biblical, spiritual, or counseling insight and these questions test the student's ability to deduce, assimilate, and otherwise process a number of factors to answer the questions.

Completion requirements are as follows:

Sections: The course is divided into several sections of approximately 50 questions each. It is not necessary to complete all sections in one setting. However, you must complete a section before submitting your work. DO NOT submit a section that is partially complete.

1. What is the core of Christ-based Counseling?

2. How many constituents comprise the process?

3. What is the first step in the Process of Being Made Whole?

4. Where is the foundation of Christ-based Counseling's effectiveness?

5. Who are the only persons who can avail themselves to CBC?

6. What must persons do first, who do not know the Lord?

7. According to Jesus, what is necessary for any person who desires a therapy where faith is involved?

8. What is the second step in the Process of Being Made Whole?

9. What is the therapy for right thinking?

10. Read the referenced text (Matt. 4:5-7).

11. Satan wants Jesus to prove that He (Jesus) is the son of God. What does Satan use as the "authority" to convince Jesus that his (Satan's) request is legitimate? (Hint: Satan makes a reference to it in verse 6,"for it ...")

12. What does Jesus use as His "authority" responding to Satan's request?

13. What verse in Scripture does Satan attempt to misuse?

14. What does Christ-based Counseling rely on?

15. What is the third step in the Process that counselees must possess?

16. What must counselees believe in the third step?

17. Name the four different types of hearers?

18. Read Mark 4:13-20, which of the hearers has God's Word snatched before it can take root in the heart?

19. Which of the hearers receives God's word, but "gives-up" upon experiencing difficulties as the result of obeying God's Word?

20. What are the characteristics of the Thorns & Thistles hearer?

21. Who believes in spite of the circumstances?

22. According to this step, the more a person believes and applies God's Word, the more...? (Complete the sentence/thinking)

23. Write the fourth step.

24. How much did the widow in the text give in life's value? (Hint: not monetary value)

25. What is ironic about our culture concerning lifestyle change?

26. What does the Process require?

27. What is the fifth step in the Process?

28. Read Mark 8:1-3. How long were the people with Jesus?

29. What physical necessity did Jesus recognize?

30. What is used as an example of completing a practical matter?

31. What is the final step in the Process?

32. Read John 15:3-9. What verb does Jesus repeat several times during the reading?

33. What will counselees be willing to do?

34. What makes most issues problematical?

35. Name two functions counselees must observe.

36. What additional therapeutic dimension is extremely important?

37. Are most problems resolved in a short timeframe?

38. Do many believers have a daily and concentrated prayer regimen?

39. What do most life changes require?

40. Name two factors necessary to reach a lifestyle change.

41. What number is used so often in the Bible that it is clearly more than a coincident?

42. What other numbers are seen often in the Bible?

43. What must believers be cautious about concerning numbers?

44. After sin, what is apparent concerning the timeframe of about forty days?

45. What is meant by the term, "Angels are purveyors of God's will?"

46. What specifically do angels accomplish?

47. Where do angels work?

48. What has God connected to their operation?

49. How many references to angels are in the Bible?

50. Why do angels refer to days in the Bible (e.g., Dan. 10:13)?

51. Events in the Bible involving "forty" refer to the completion of a _____, _____, or _____. (Fill in blanks)

52. If the principle concerning "forty" is true, how many times should it be shown in the Bible?

53. What happens in Genesis 7:12?

54. What happens in Numbers 13:25?

55. What happens in Deuteronomy 10:10?

56. What happens in I Kings 19:5-8?

57. What was the prophet instructed to do in Ezekiel 4:6?

58. How many days did it take the angel to arrive upon Daniel's request?

59. Was the angel's mission over when He arrived to Daniel?

60. How long do you think it would take for the angel to complete the mission? Why?

61. How long did Nineveh have to repent in Jonah 3:4?

62. Are there more than two or three references to the use of forty days in the Bible? (Shown in the questions above)

63.	Where is the precedent found for the principle concerning forty days?

64.	More importantly, give two examples in the New Testament where the forty-day principle is evident.

65.	Who was on the scene in both cases?

66.	What is one of the most important characteristics of prayer in Luke 11:5-8; and Luke18:1-8?

67.	In Luke 11:5-8, what does the man desire from his neighbor?

68.	Was his original request provided?

69.	Given his neighbor's original response, how did the man respond?

70.	Recall, what is Jesus' topic in Luke 11:5-8?

71.	What is the primary characteristic Jesus teaches about prayer in verses 5-8?

72.	Who are the two characters in Luke 18:1-8?

73.	Concerning prayer, what is Jesus' specific objective for believers in verse 1?

74.	How was the widow's initial request received by the judge?

75.	What type of character did the judge possess?

76.	How did the widow respond to the judge's initial response to her request?

77.	Eventually, how does the judge respond to the widow's request?

78.   What is the primary characteristic Jesus is teaching us by the parable of the woman before the unjust judge?

79.   What two terms does Paul use concerning prayer?

80.   Read Matthew 17:14-21. Who was ill?

81.   What was the symptoms of the boy's illness?

82.   Who tried to cure the boy?

83.   Why were they unsuccessful?

84.   Explain what Jesus meant by His explanation for the disciples inability to cure the boy?

85.   What do the most challenging issues in life require?

86.   What must be demonstrated, persistently?

87.   When believers have a consistent prayer discipline, who is waiting for marching orders from the Lord?

88.   Believers must not worship or pray to what beings?

89.   What did Jesus know concerning the angelic dimension?

90.   Angelic success is often connected to our _____ (fill in space).

91.   Read Ephesians 6:10-20. What does Paul make clear?

92.   Once the "overwhelming objective" is accomplished, what is cleared?

93.   What type of weaponry does Paul address?

94.   What are the focal verses in Ephesians Chapter 6 for PBMW?

95.   What do verses 16-18 highlight?

96.   What else does Paul add?

97.   What can God do in a single day?

98.   What is required for most matters requiring spiritual intervention?

99.   What other term is also noteworthy? Concerning God and angels is there any difference between the two?

100.   When believers pray in a range of forty days, what will they experience?

101.   Will issues always be resolved in forty days? Explain. Where does the additional five days come from?

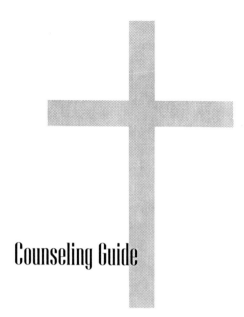

Counseling Guide

Block 1

1. What percentage of the population is obese or overweight?

2. How many deaths are attributed to obesity each year?

3. Concerning food, what are the three issues?

4. What were some of the bodily differences experienced by the author he noted during a fast?

5. Who directed that believers maintain their typical functions and disposition when fasting?

6. What is the focus of most weight management programs?

7. Stated simply, what is the bottom line of weight management?

8. What is the important factor often neglected?

9. Give some examples of the full scope on fasting in the Bible?

10. What do persons who have conducted Biblical research on fasting usually find?

11. Biblically, where is the first fast as we know it?

12. Who fasted in the first fast, and how long was it?

13. Who are the other persons who fasted at least forty days?

14. What does the author name a fast representing a period when God leads a person or people into a transition?

15. According to many writers, what should be the objective of fasting?

16. What do most writers frown about concerning fasting?

17. Based on their illustrations, what types of dire conditions exist, which lead a person to fast?

18. Do spiritual matters only represent spiritual goals? Explain.

19. Are issues in believer's life purely spiritual?

20. What does the spiritual realm affect?

21. Why do people pray and exhibit faith?

22. What do people desire when they pray?

23. What surprised the author?

24. Where is the beginning or the principal cause for fasting found?

25. What is it that we rarely recognize about Genesis Chapter 3?

26. How many times is eating shown in the first 19 verses of Genesis 3?

27. How often is eat or other forms of the word found in the curses representing the man in Genesis 3:17-19?

28. Concerning the fruit's origin of growth, what became cursed when the man ate the fruit?

29. What will be at least three outcomes of man's sin concerning food?

30. Prior to sin, is it stated or implied that food is necessary to sustain life?

31. Before sin occurred why was eating undertaken?

32. Explain why the serpent's lure was so appealing to the woman?

33. What are the three characteristics the woman perceived about the forbidden fruit?

34. What is the problem if a person believes that food was necessary to sustain life before sin occurred?

35. Although man had not sinned yet, was sin represented in man's environment?

36. Prior to man committing sin, did humanity live under the authority of death?

37. Concerning life, which tree seems to be required for living?

38. Prior to sin, did the man and woman have to eat from the tree of life to live? Explain.

39. Concerning food, what did the curses do?

40. Since the ground is cursed. What else is cursed?

41. What contributes to the dying process?

42. Why did God curse food, which was designed for man's pleasure?

43. Explain three critical areas in Genesis where eating is the topic or cause?

44. What should happen once the believer understands the Biblical insights about food?

46. Where do most of the illustrations of fasting occur in the Bible? Give examples.

47. Is fasting also found in the New Testament? Give examples.

48. Who must be the center focus concerning fasting?

49. As Jesus is preparing to launch into His earthly ministry, what does he do for forty days?

50. Why does the counselor call it an extended fast?

Block 2

51. What is the length of the majority of fasts found in the Bible?

52. What kind of fast did Jesus practice?

53. What are the purposes for the fasts Jesus experienced?

54. According to Matthew 4:2, when did Jesus become hungry?

55. Who is on the scene?

56. Where was this being on the scene previously?

57. What was Jesus' first recorded temptation?

58. What is ironic about Jesus' first temptation?

59. What was Jesus reply to Satan's temptation?

60. Concerning "live," generically, what could one conclude by Jesus' answer?

61. However, in the context of the question and Jesus condition of hunger, what did Jesus mean?

62. Obviously, what does man also live by?

63. Was Jesus fast only concerning his spiritual preparation? Explain.

64. What did Jesus know the facts about?

65. While we must eat, what does eating do if it is not controlled?

66. While there are numerous spiritual advantages, what does Jesus also teach about fasting?

67. What is a striking image for us today?

68. What is it that most believers do not realize?

69. Based on the effect of sin, what did man move from and to concerning his diet?

70. When did man begin eating animals?

71. With a few exceptions, what was the basic framework for eating animals?

72. What was to be avoided?

73. Was animal consumption a part of man's original design? Explain.

74. Apparently, what happened that caused man to begin eating animals?

75. Concerning man's life expectancy, what happens after the flood?

76. Do you think his new life expectancy has anything to do with animal consumption?

77. Does the Bible have a view of persons with uncontrolled appetites?

78. What is comparable to gluttony?

79. How does the counselor view the condition of the typical person in our culture?

80. Based on CDC statistics, and personal observations, how often and where does the typical person eat?

81. What accusation did Jesus face?

82. What was the term used to label him?

83. Today, how is this term used?

84. According to Paul, what does he warn about in Romans 14:20?

85. What was his purpose for warning about eating meat found in vs. 21?

86. While food offered to idols was the topic, what did Paul say about our God in Corinthians 8:4-8?

87. Should we confuse Paul's statements concerning food offered to idols with the origin of food as sustenance? Explain.

88. Is food extraordinarily cursed because it is offered to idols?

89. Does Paul's warning to the Corinthians discuss the basic truth about food in general?

90. What were Paul's instructions to Timothy concerning?

91. In Timothy 4:1-3, what are some of the false teachers forbidding and commanding?

92. Does the clause abstaining from meats have anything to do with fasting?

93. How is every creature sanctified for food?

94. Again, how or what do you believe this meat has been offered to before consumption?

95. Since this meat offered to idols is set apart for food, are there any spiritual or sin implications?

96. What is the source of the body's nutritional strength?

97. What is much more profitable to our body wellness than physical efforts?

98. According to I Timothy 4:7-8, how does physical exercise compare to principles of faith?

99. How is godliness profitable?

100. Paul is speaking of both... (Complete the sentence)

Block 3

101. What does Paul state in I Timothy 4:8 that affirms godliness' relationship to physical and spiritual wellness?

102. While exercise and proper diet have obvious benefit, what is even more important to body wellness?

103. What issues lead the way concerning God's Word related to physical wellness?

104. What is a multi-billion dollar industry in the United States?

105. What are some of the quick methods of earning money from those desiring to control food consumption?

106. In your opinion, do believers pray about most issues concerning wellness?

107. What is a novel idea?

108. Consumption control is related to… (Complete the sentence)

109. What does Paul call the body?

110. Who do our physical bodies glorify?

111. What does our physical health relate to directly?

112. Are there denominations that do not support fasting?

113. Why are there believers who do not believe that fasting is a principle to be exercised today?

114. Is fasting a major theme in books such as Romans, Corinthians, and Colossians?

115. Was fasting a factor when the Church was launched?

116. Does Paul mention fasting at all? If so, what book in the Bible?

117. Why does the author believe that Jesus intended for fasting to be a discipline in the believer's life?

118. What might the term, "those days" mean to some people?

119. Why is this view defeated?

120. What period is fasting relevant?

121. What else does Jesus seem to indicate about fasting during this period?

122. Viewing the analogy in Luke 5:36-38, Mark 9:14, and Mark 2:18, what seems to be the relationship to fasting?

123. Contextually, what is this new and expanded purpose?

124. In comparison, what was the view under the Law?

125. What is the other experience in the disciples' life that underscored this new and expanded purpose for fasting?

126. When the disciples could not heal the boy, what did the disciples ask Jesus?

127. What was Jesus reply to the disciples' question?

128. Did Jesus mean that when they saw the boy they should have prayed and fasted immediately?

129. What does fasting provide when coupled with prayer?

130. What is the point concerning fasting in the believer's life?

131. However, our love for food consumption is so pervasive, what is it that we do not like?

132. What is one of the least likely Christian necessities a believer will practice?

133. Similar to Jesus, what is it that persons who fast experience regularly?

134. The more a person fasts, what does the person build?

135. What does the body begin to do?

136. How is the "psycho-addictive" nature of eating overcome?

137. What does the term "psycho-addictive" mean in terms of fasting?

138. What are some of the manifestations of fasting?

139. What must believers understand about fasting?

140. The more a person fasts, what does the body begin to do?

141. Whose approval must a person seek about fasting?

142. Recognizing that obesity significantly reduces life expectancy, what alternative are people choosing?

143. What is the net effect of these drastic procedures?

144. What does this demonstrate relative to trying to diet?

145. What can have the same result as major surgeries?

146. What happens after fasting three or more days?

147. What is the power element combined with fasting?

148. What is extremely powerful?

149. What may be the decisive factor? Why?

150. Why will some people succeed where they could not with dieting alone?

Block 4

151. What is also important to couple with fasting?

152. What does a person maintain while fasting?

153. What else is combined with Christ-based Consumption Control?

154. What did Jesus mean when he explained the need for prayer and fasting?

155. What do people with an established prayer life have?

156. What also should believers establish?

157. What does the counselor recommend for a person who is establishing a fast pattern?

158. If it is not possible to fast for 7 days, what should the believer do?

159. What is the 3+3+1 method?

160. What is recommended for people who are extremely weight challenge?

161. Why is an extended fast well worth it?

162. Who must be consulted before embarking on any fast?

163. What will happen when the believer resumes eating after a fast?

164. When fasting, where is the battle going to be?

165. What should a person drink during a fast to control food consumption?

166. What is more of an issue than starvation or food depravation?

167. When hunger arises, how should the believer respond?

168. Once the believer completes a full week, how should the believer follow-up?

169. Results depend on... (Complete sentence)

170. What does the counselor recommend as the day for beginning the fast?

171. What will happen if a believer maintains the weekly fast schedule?

172. Concerning caloric intake, what is the reduction in calories?

173. What is the caloric reduction for a person who fasts for forty days based on 2000 calories a day?

174. After each fast, whether short or long, if the believer combines this with dieting, how might you describe the reduction?

175. What is possible as a believer builds the fast threshold?

176. What are some of the results after the first week or seven days of fasting?

177. Since weight loss is slower, what is very valuable?

178. How long should a person wait before considering dramatic weight loss?

179. What is evidence of faith and resolve?

180. Will all the weight gained over a period of years be removed in forty days? Explain.

181. What must a believer's mind be convinced to do?

182. There is a lot of misinformation about...? (Complete the sentence)

183. What is going to be required for a person who does not eXaltorcise at all?

184. What may it require for a person who has an exercise routine?

185. How many minutes should a person eXaltorcise for weight control?

186. Why should there be substantial motivation for an eXaltorcise program?

187. What do some believers do two or three times a day?

188. Concerning the heart, what does eXaltorcise require?

189. While helpful, what may not contribute to weight loss?

190. How must a person walk in order to get the advantage of burning a higher level of calories?

191. Who can have difficulty exercising?

192. Give examples of physical problems eXaltorcise can cause?

193. What is one of the best vehicles for persons with excessive weight?

194. Concerning listening or watching entertainment, what is of primary importance?

195. What is the problem with people who want to read as they go through their routine?

196. What is an immediate and added incentive for an exercise program?

197. What does Dr. Kenneth Cooper affirm?

198. Can this be an alternative to medicinal therapy for hypertension?

199. Who should persons consult if he/she desires to control hypertension with physical eXaltorcise?

200. What does the term good shape mean often?

Block 5

201. Does a slim or small frame mean a person is in good shape?

202. How is "good shape" determined?

203. Concerning exercise, what do some people prefer as opposed to aerobic exercise?

204. Does a muscular physique mean a person is in good shape?

205. Why do some people prefer isometric exercise activities?

206. Why must persons with hypertension be cautious about isometric exercise according to Cooper?

207. What approach does the counselor use personally?

208. Can anyone assume he/she will not have a heart attack or stroke?

209. What term does the medical community use concerning the likelihood of a medical event?

210. Who has some degree of risk?

211. What increases the risk of a major stroke, heart attack, and related illnesses?

212. When dieting contributes to weight loss, does this necessarily improve the health profile?

213. What is the trade-off with an Atkins type diet?

214. Although it is successful with some people, what is a major concern about meat/protein diets?

215. What is the purpose of consumption control/weight management?

216. Does the Bible support eating high animal meat content as a daily staple?

217. Why will some people find fasting more hassle free than dieting?

218. What is typically lower in calories when compared to food?

219. How is both fasting and dieting similar?

220. One person fasts for weight management, and another diets. Who is more likely to consume more calories than planned?

Weight Deficit Disorders
A Christ-based Counseling Perspective

No counseling guide on weight management would be complete without addressing anorexia and bulimia. Here, these are characterized as Weight Deficit Disorders (WDD). Statistically, these disorders are not the dominant weight issues in the nation today. Nevertheless, they are life-threatening conditions. Certainly, there is a distinction between the two, but the point is that the level of weight is dangerously low.

Typical Causes and Therapy

The typical causes considered by eating disorder specialists are varied. As usual with most disorders, specialists consider a number of causative factors (e.g., genetics, environment, self-image, stresses, etc.). Depending on the severity, in-patient care may be required. Some type of psychotherapy is also recommended. It is not unusual when other opportunistic disorders accompany the eating disorder (bi-polar, panic, etc.). Therefore, psychotropic drugs may also be a part of the therapy.

The Cause, a Christ-based Counseling Perspective

The Christ-based Counseling model offers an insightful view of the causative "condition" at some level in the WDD counselee. If it is determined that there is not a pathological purpose (i.e., malfunctioning organs), then the Christ-based analysis provides the likely framework for understanding the root cause of weight deficit disorders. This same analysis is provided in the Christ-based Counseling Model in the Hard Core Cases section. First, a brief view of mankind is beneficial.

"Quadmetric" View of Man

There are a number of different views of what constitutes the human organism. Some believe that man is a dichotomy. That is, man is body and soul. Some hold a position that man is tripartite. Man is body, soul, and spirit. There is Biblical support for both of these. However, I believe the most definitive finding about man was revealed by Jesus. Jesus was engaged in a conversation when a religious man asked about the most important commandment. Jesus' reply helps us understand the intricacies of man:

And thou shalt love the Lord thy God with all thy heart, and with all thy soul, and with all thy mind, and with all thy strength: this is the first commandment (Mark 12:30, KJV)

Note, there are four distinct characteristics of mankind which are involved in demonstrating love toward God. These four functions within man must demonstrate a certain standard. Love is the standard or metric. This is the origin of the term, "quadmetric" view. Jesus' first instruction is to love God with the heart. Obviously, the physical heart is not where love can reside. Jesus means to love God with our spirit. This spirit, which Jesus references is different than the Holy Spirit. Jesus likely means that a person's disposition, demeanor, or behavior pattern should represent a love and reverence for God. While it exceeds the scope of this book, there is no doubt that one's spirit is at the core of a persons disposition. Secondly, Jesus speaks of loving God with all of one's soul. The soul is the seat of emotions. The person who loves God does so with an emotional response that is consistent with the truths in God's Word. Thirdly, loving God with the mind involves the cognitive process. This is where thinking occurs. Thinking is based on God's Word as opposed to the world's system or logic. Finally, loving God with all of one's strength. This appears to be physical, but it is also all encompassing. Loving with all of one's strength involves what the believer does, where the believer goes, how the believer acts and more.

Once the religious leader repeated and affirmed what Jesus stated, verse 34 discloses the following:

And when Jesus saw that he answered discreetly, he said unto him, Thou art not far from the kingdom of God. And no man after that durst ask him any question
(Mark 12:33, KJV)

While the specific topic of discussion involved the most important commandment, we are able to deduce from the statement the four parts of mankind. The text further shows that the man answered discreetly. This an affirmation of the detailed parts of man as well as the principal commandment.

As shown above the heart can also be rendered behavior pattern. Human beings are self-gratification oriented. Treasures, which offer great satisfaction are the ones that dominate the behavior.

Jesus instructed his followers about an inherent quality of human beings. People are self-gratification oriented (Matthew 10:39; 16:25). The instruments or objects of self-gratification can be identified as treasures. These treasures can exist in any form including material possessions, objects, lifestyles, habits, social status, position, emotional behavior, relationships, etc. (Matthew 19:16-22).

All of a person's energies are directed toward these treasures, which in-turn fulfills one's drive for self-gratification. Ironically, an individual may even understand or be aware of the depravity and/or danger of his or her condition. Nevertheless, the behavior does not cease to provide some degree of satisfaction (i.e., comfort, defense, notoriety, e.g.).

These extremely desperate situations can only be understood in the same context as someone who is suffering from congestive heart failure. The Christ-based Counseling model refers to these as Hard-Core conditions. This is when a person's life is completely dominated by this condition, and the activities will literally lead to death.

As stated earlier the behavior, act, event, or objects can be identified as treasures, which offer some degree of gratification. However, these treasures are merely manifestations of the counselee's spiritual condition.

Jesus, who already possesses a complete analysis of the Hard Core condition, provides the remedy so that the Christ-based specialist can move directly to the "heart" of the matter. He states, "where your treasures are there will your heart be also (Matthew 6:21)."

In short, these "treasures" are assigned an extremely high priority. In fact, these treasures become as meaningful as life itself. Therefore, the WDD counselee will not cease unhealthy behavior. These and many others are seeking their treasures which in-turn provides a sense of self-gratification as bizarre and twisted as it may seem.

Notwithstanding why the behavior occurs (e.g., fear, harmful experience, defense mechanism, self-image, peer pressure, similar factors), God's Word in Jesus Christ provides the explanation, and His Word provides the approach.

Program Framework, CBC, The Process of Being Made Whole

The "Process of Making Whole" is as effective with Hard-Core counseling cases as with the cases, which are more typical (marital, parental, emotional, etc.). Remember, Christ-based Counseling works in the physical and spiritual realms to assure change.

Along with medical support (e.g., physical, psychiatric), several steps should be taken to assist the counselee in overcoming Hard-Core (i.e., WDD) or any other related problems:

1. The counselee needs an explanation of the depth of his or her condition. It has been described here.

2. The counselee must recognize that some degree of gratification is being experienced by his or her behavior. Again, gratification can exist in several forms.
3. The counselee must re-examine the depth of his or her relationship to living as a believer.
4. Christian virtues must replace the counselee's treasures. The counselee must view life from God's perspective, particularly in regards to priorities. However, this will not occur until the counselee "sacrifices" his or her own treasures for heavenly ones (Matt. 9:21-22).
5. The counselee needs a long-term support group were meetings are held regularly.
6. A timeline must be monitored to highlight periods when the hard-core behavior is repeated.
7. As the counselee surpasses milestones or goals, some form of recognition should be acknowledged.
8. A rigorous study and consistent regimen of CBC exercises (see The Process of Being Made Whole) should be entered. These studies would involve assurances of faith, trust, prayer, fellowship, spirit-based esteem, perseverance, and God's provisions for the counselee.
9. As shown in the Process of Being Made Whole, the counselee must keep in mind that overcoming the WDD will require a combination of time and consistent CBC activities.

Progress Assessment and Maxim

If the counselee does not experience any detectable progress over a period (e.g., one year), then the counselor must examine the counselee's confession of faith. Is the counselee truly "born-again?"

If the counselee is born again (John 3:7), AND the counselee has allowed God's Word to take root in his or her heart (Matt. 13:23), AND the counselee confesses the depravity of his or her acts (John 8:10-11; Luke 7:37-38, 47-48, 50), it is impossible for the counselee to remain in the same condition with the same level of self-deprecating behavior. There is not one Biblical principle to support the coexistence of long-term depravity (i.e. sin) and the spiritually born-again believer.

Weight Deficit Disorders Thumbnail Assessment (Master)

Assessment Instructions: This assessment is an indicator of whether or not the counselee is suffering with a WDD. Since every person can be so unique, all of the questions should be considered in making a determination. The rationale is provided for each question.

1. How often do you think about food?
   [Persons suffering with WDD are obsessed with food. That is, how to avoid consumption of food.]

2. Do you exercise? ____ If so, how much
   [Persons suffering with WDD "may" obsess on exercise. However, it is also possible that the person exercises very little.]
   ☐ Once weekly
   ☐ Twice weekly
   ☐ Three times weekly
   ☐ Four or more times a week

3. Name your close friends?
   [Typically, persons suffering with a WDD are not popular. There may be a person or two at best who would be considered close friends.]

4. How often do you see or speak with your close friends?
   [This is a follow-up question to determine how close the counselee is to the persons identified in question 3.]

5. If you have siblings, where are you in order of age (e.g., oldest, youngest, etc.)?
   [This question simply establishes whether there are other persons in the family, and where the counselee is in the age order.]

6. Any other persons with weight deficit disorders in your family?
   [Often, other family members also experience WDD]

7. Do you eat in front of others?
   [Some WDD specialists observe that counselees do not like eating with others.]

8. Please describe your current therapy if any for this condition?
   [Record whether the counselee is attending another therapist]

9. Physically, how would you describe your characteristics
   [It is not unusual for the WDD counselee to feel that he/she is fat, and unattractive. This rationale applies to questions 10 and 11.]

   ☐ I'm gorgeous
   ☐ I am nice looking
   ☐ I'm o.k.
   ☐ I'm unattractive

10. When you think of your weight, what best describes you?

       ☐ I'm very fat
       ☐ I'm fat
       ☐ I'm about the same as others my age and size
       ☐ I'm thin

11. Name the top five foods you enjoy eating?
[Attempt to identify food the counselee enjoys. Where possible, these should be a part of a three times per day, forty-day eating covenant.

12. Do you have regular bouts of regurgitating what you eat?
[Whereas the anorexic does not eat regularly, the bulimic has a practice of regurgitating.]

13. How much does the counselee weigh? _____
[Is the counselee's weight below the norm?]

Weight Deficit Disorders Thumbnail Assessment

1. How often do you think about food?

2. Do you exercise? ___ If so, how much

   ☐ Once weekly
   ☐ Twice weekly
   ☐ Three times weekly
   ☐ Four or more times a week

3. Name your close friends?

4. How often do you see your close friends?

5. If you have siblings, where are you in order of age (e.g., oldest, youngest, etc.)?

6. Any other persons with weight deficit disorders in your family?

7. Do you eat in front of others?

8. Please describe your current therapy if any for this condition?

9. Physically, how would you describe your characteristics

    ☐ I'm gorgeous
    ☐ I am nice looking
    ☐ I'm o.k.
    ☐ I'm unattractive

10. When you think of your weight, what best describes you?

    ☐ I'm very fat
    ☐ I'm fat
    ☐ I'm about the same as others my age and size
    ☐ I'm thin

11. Name the top five foods you enjoy eating?

12. Do you have regular bouts of regurgitating what you eat?

13. How much do you weigh?

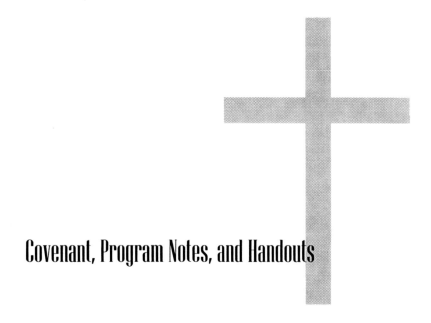

Covenant, Program Notes, and Handouts

The Power of the CBWM Covenant

More than one-hundred and fifty persons were involved in the Christ-based Weight Management project. I have discovered that one of the critical success factors is the Christ-based Weight Management Covenant.

The CBWM covenant ensures that the believer studies the principles, and stays on course for periods of 45 days or more throughout a year. Thereafter, the covenant is renewed as needed. The persons can readjust the schedule every forty-five days. If we were only trying to manage weight, forty-five days would be enough for many participants. Once the weight goal is reached, the covenant could be terminated. However, much more is at stake. Most of the participants are trying to overcome the shackles and authority food has over their lives. If they do not stay in the program, it is not long before they gravitate back to their old ways.

The Covenant Principle is equally liberating when it is applied to our circumstances over time. It is very convicting and powerful. I have found that it is the most feared part of the program for participants. However, the covenant's effectiveness cannot be argued.

It is the sign of the most determined and committed person. Moreover, it is rewarded with God's riches blessings when He is involved. After all, He started the Covenant Principle, and this is the reason why it is a critical success factor for persons in the CBWM program.

When did He start the covenant process? A covenant is an agreement between two parties or more. It is similar to a contract. However, there is a significant difference. Biblically speaking, a contract is based on law, but a covenant is based on love. God initiated the first covenant. It is commonly called the Edenic Covenant. It is not coincidental that "eating" was involved in the first covenant.

There were two parties in the covenant, God and man. God gave man full reign and authority over the elements of the earth. It was understood that God presented it to man, and God would perpetuate it for man. Man's part was to do as he pleased with the earth. Keep in mind that whatever man pleased was going to be pleasing to God. There was only one "do not." "And the Lord God commanded the man saying, of every tree of the garden thou mayest freely eat: But of the tree of the knowledge of good and evil, thou shalt not eat of it for in the day that thou eatest thereof thou shalt surely die." Genesis 2:16-17 KJV.

The rest is history. The first covenant involved eating. No wonder a covenant designed to overcome our obsession and addiction to food is so feared. We love God to commit to us and bless us. However, we shrink when it comes to making a covenant with Him for our benefit -- until we get in trouble. God began the process, and Christ-based Weight Management incorporates the covenant principle as a major success factor.

Understanding the Program's Design

Remember that our dietary habits are years old (e.g., 20 or more years). Participants need to implement the principles for at least forty-five days to establish one's personal faithfulness in the spiritual realm.

This should be understood as the beginning of a lifestyle change. As with prayer, obedience, and other biblical principles, some aspect of fasting and food abstinence should remain in the believer's life for the rest of his or her days. Therefore, milestone dates are 45, 90, 180,

270, and 360 days from the first day of the program as follows: Enter here the day you started the program ____/____/_____ Weight: _____

    45 Days to Glory: ___/___/___   Weight: _____
    90 Days of Promise: ___/___/___   Weight: _____
    180 Days of Determination: ___/___/___   Weight: _____
    270 Days of Certainty: ___/___/___   Weight: _____
    The Year of Celebration: ___/___/___   Weight: _____

Discipline and Consistency: It is highly recommended that you stay on the scheduled commitment for the period agreed in this covenant unless there is an emergency or other reason necessitating a change. Please confer with the witnesses of the covenant, or the program administrator before modifying your program. It is also recommended that you do not begin your weekly Christ-based fast any later than Monday. Initial ____

A Promise with the Community of Believers and the God we serve: Do not take this covenant lightly. This covenant represents a spiritual promise. It is better not to make the covenant than to make it and violate it. If you must discontinue use the guidelines under Discipline and Consistency to modify or discontinue your vow. Initial _____

Faith Accountability Disclaimer: I personally have heard and participated in the Christ-based Weight Management program. I willingly participate and make this commitment based on my own faith and personal conviction. I was not forced, coerced, or otherwise manipulated to participate in this program. I desire this program for my own personal well-being. I realize that any program addressing issues of weight, food consumption, diet, or any other health maintenance activities (e.g., medication, surgery, physical therapy, etc.) have risks. I accept any known or unknown risks. I have been informed to **check with my physician** concerning the principles in the program. Should any physical or terminal condition occur whether related or unrelated to this program, none of the parties shall be held responsible including officers or members of _____, Pastor/Elder/Bishop/Dr. _____, _____, or any organization she/he represents. I am thankful for the opportunity to be involved in this program. Initial _____

Establishing Your Christ-based Fast Pattern

You should determine how many days a week you will live "physically" on the Word of God for solid food.

Here are the recommended schedules:

- Spiritual growth and Extreme Weight loss (75 lbs or more) 4 or more days
- Spiritual growth and Significant Weight loss (25 lbs -75 lbs) 4 days
- Spiritual growth and Moderate Weight loss (10 lbs to 20 lbs.): 3 days
- Spiritual growth and Maintenance: 2 days

Example of Actual Schedules with a Monday 12:01 am Start:

Determined Disciple's Fast (Aggressive weight loss program)

4 days per week (Monday through Thursday after 4:00 p.m.):

The final meal will be on Sunday and the fast ends the following Thursday at 4:00 pm.

Level II Fast (Normal weight loss program)

4 days per week (2 halves):

1st Half: The final meal will be on Sunday, and the fast ends Monday night 11:59 p.m.
Tuesday is an open day.
2nd half Fasting begins Wednesday 12:01 am and ends Friday 4:00 pm
Saturday open
Sunday open

Level III Fast (Extended weight loss program)

4.5 days

1st Half: The final meal will be on Sunday 11:59 p.m., and the fast ends Tuesday at 4:00 p.m.

Wednesday is an open day.

2nd Half: The final meal is Wednesday night at 11:59 p.m., and the fast ends Friday at 4:00 p.m.

½ day: Saturday 12:01 a.m. to 12:01 p.m.

Level IV Options (Varying degrees of weight loss desired). This level is designed to build the fast threshold and move to a more progressive level at a later date.

Option 1) Final meal on Sunday. Next meal 4:00 p.m. on Tuesday.

Wednesday open

Fast continues 12:01 am on Thursday. Next meal 4 p.m. on Friday

Saturday open

Sunday open until 11:59 p.m.

Option 2) Final meal on Sunday. Next meal 4:00 p.m. Tuesday.

All other days are open.

Option 3) Final meal on Sunday. Next meal on Tuesday morning or thereafter. All other days are open.

Note: It is highly recommended that you stay on the scheduled commitment for the first 45 day periods before making any change. Establishing discipline is imperative. It is also recommended that you do not begin your weekly fast any later than Monday.

Weighing to Manage Your Weight:

NOTICE: The first weigh-in is 6 days after you begin the program. You will not be weighing again until you conclude the first 45 days. Obsessive weighing can be very discouraging. This is a faith-based program. Measure your success by the degree you honor your covenant.

Once you conclude your first forty-five days, it is important that you always weigh yourself on the morning of the day you conclude your fast.

If you split your fast with two fast periods during the week, you weigh on the last day of the second fast period.

Managing Weight Results: If you find that your weight is up, then fast an additional day or more. This is how you will keep your weight in check. If your weight is consistent with the weight of your last weigh-in, then continue your program as usual.

Understanding Plateaus: Depending on the amount of weight you desire to loose, there will be a series of periods when you will plateau. This means you could go several weeks without seeing reduction results. **STAY ON YOUR PROGRAM**. During these periods, you need to focus on the other benefits of a Christ-based program. Faith—by definition—assumes that it does not appear that anything is happening. Do not be fooled. This is why prayer is so important. Once you have concluded the current covenant period, you can make any adjustments you think is necessary for your next covenant period.

RECOMMENDATION: It is better to be less aggressive early. Choose a Level IV Option, and do more than required by your covenant if you feel particularly strong and confident. You can exceed your covenant each week if you desire. However, if you have a strong constitution, you can be aggressive. Fasts that last three or more consecutive days are the most effective. If you need to loose more than fifty pounds, be prepared to give yourself a year or more to loose the weight. A year is recommended for everyone regardless of one's weight profile. There are persons who have definitely reached the fifty-pound goal in less than six months. Do not forget to eXaltorcise regularly -- at least four times a week. This is very necessary to burn the sugars and other contents generated from drinking the various juices among other benefits.

Hierarchy of Acceptable CBWM Fluids

Preferred
    Juices, 100%
    Water
    Vitamins (multi and specific)
    Breadth mints

Alternative (no more than twice per day, or 20 oz.)
    Smoothies (without pulp)

Juice Drinks (10% or more of fruit juice)
Slim Fast
Ensure and similar drinks
Non-caffeinated chocolate

Only if you must:
Sodas, and other drinks
Coffee, Tea

For diabetics with physician's approval:
Broths
Jello
Soups without meat (e.g., tomato, pea, bean, potato, etc.), nuts

Be sure to check regularly with your physician where any pre-existing condition exists (e.g., diabetes, hypertension, etc.); and check with your physician before beginning any program including eXaltorcise and consumption control.

Christ-based Weight Management Covenant

Dear Lord,
   This covenant is between me, You, and the believers who sign this covenant below. I enter this covenant willfully. I understand that this program is for my spiritual growth, and physical health. I promise that I will use this program to glorify you. Excluding any serious illnesses, grave family event, or similar crisis, I will stay on this program for a year from _____ to _____. If for any reason I am unable to continue due to some unforeseen event, I will resume the balance of the scheduled program as soon as possible. Your Word instructs me to keep a promise (Ecclesiastes 5:5, Matthew 5:33-37). I know you see and know everything. I also know that it is not Your will that anything should master or dominate my life other than You. I know it is your will for me to overcome any obsession, bondage, or enslavement to food (I Corinthians 6:12-13). Therefore, I know you hear me, and you are completely with me in this effort (1 John 5:15). **Lord, if I reach my weight goal before one year, it is still necessary to keep some aspect of food abstinence in my life. I will select a program from Level IV at that time.**
   I know how important it is to submit willfully to Your will for my life.

Therefore, I promise to perform the seven activities. I do this before You, and the Christian community. The fasting and abstinence pattern that I promise to do is (Place an X by one below):

☐ Determined Disciples Fast (Aggressive weight loss program)
☐ Level II Fast (Normal weight loss program)
☐ Level III (Extended weight loss program)
☐ Level IV Options

I will contact the CBWM minister or counselor of record concerning any questions or concerns.

Your Servant and Child Eternally,

_____
Signature

Witnessed by (Matthew 18:16):

_____   _____   _____
Signature   Signature   Signature

Please submit the original of this covenant to the CBWM counselor or minister for your folder.
    Congratulatory issued after first six days

Praise God and Congratulations!

    You have made it through the most difficult part of the Seven Days of Heaven. Bless the Lord! Spiritually, you are being powered by the Word of God and the Word's influence on your life. Physically, momentum and experience are also on your side. You have demonstrated to yourself, your family in Christ, and the spiritual principalities (e.g., heaven's angels, angels of darkness, demons, etc.) that you are willing to make the sacrifices.
    HERE is why the angels and humans know that you are serious. You have satisfactorily satisfied several steps, which are a test of your conviction. You should have satisfactorily completed the following:

1. Process of Being Made Whole.

2. Attended the forum/seminar or attended your first counseling session.
3. Completed the first 50 questions of the Christ-based Weight Management program.
4. Completed the Seven Days of Heaven.

These are designed to teach you spiritual principles, and establish your depth of conviction and level of determination.

The next step is to establish the **permanency** of this pattern in your life.

NOW you are prepared to establish your new lifestyle as a spiritual fact, and a physical habit. This is called the Forty-Five Days to Glory. As you know from completing the Process of Being Made Whole course, it takes about 40 days to establish a new pattern in your life. Next in the program is to sign a covenant with God and two or three other witnesses/believers that you **promise and must**:

1. Establish and stay on your selected fast schedule.
2. Pray each day, and persistently ask the Lord to stay on your schedule.
3. Pray each day, persistently thanking God for giving you success.
4. Pray each day, persistently for the other persons in your group.
5. Attend one session a week at the church, on-line, or by appointment.
6. Complete at least six Christ-based Weight Management sessions.
7. eXaltorcise four days a week at least twenty or more minutes each day. (You can only eXaltorcise to Christian music, or with praises on your mind and heart. [Examples: brisk walking, praising in place with or without weights, biking, jogging, and similar activities])

Note: You can attend Monday night group sessions at church (time:_____), or on-line at (time:_____), or contact _____for individual sessions.

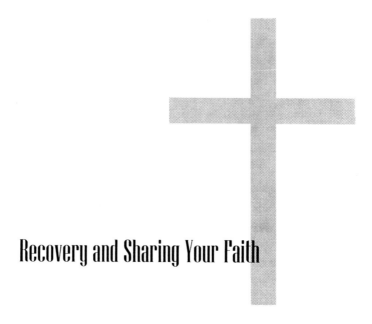

Recovery and Sharing Your Faith

Recovery

Almost everyone who begins the program has good intentions. There can be many reasons for discontinuing the program. Typically, medical issues cause participants to discontinue the program temporarily. Others simply are overwhelmed by the dominance food has over their lives. It is important to recover as soon as possible.

I recommend that persons who desire to recover simply fast a half-day, or one day per week for four weeks. The fast begins in the morning when the participant awakes, and lasts until the next day; or the fast begins in the morning when the participant awakes, and lasts until 1:00 p.m. the same day.

Once the four-week period is over, establish a new covenant or continue with a new covenant. I recommend that you use Level IV. Options 2 or 3 for forty-five days.

Sharing Your Faith

Participants find that as they begin to show results of the CBWM program, people become interested in how they are getting such results. It is so important to appropriately share one or more of the following about the program:

CBWM is based on disciplines in Jesus life.
CBWM requires an intimate relationship with Him.
CBWM is a spiritually empowered program.
CBWM requires a daily prayer life.
CBWM principles must be reviewed continuously.
CBWM is for weight maintenance, loss, or gain.
CBWM is a "rest-of-your-life" program

The Christ-based Weight Management program should never be conveyed as fasting. It is much more than fasting. If someone desires to know the Lord, you should be prepared to lead the person to Jesus Christ. There are plenty of books on this topic. If you do not have any literature or helps for leading a person to Christ, please contact the CBWM program administrator at:

Christbasedweightmanagement.org
or
CBWMprogram@aol.com.

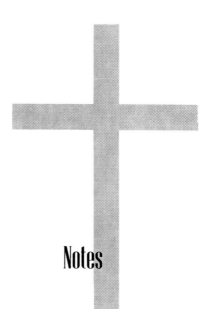

Notes

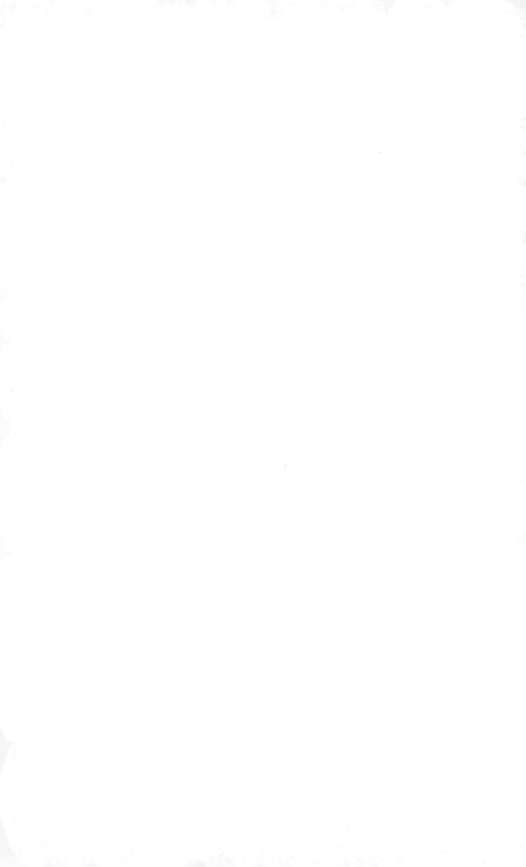

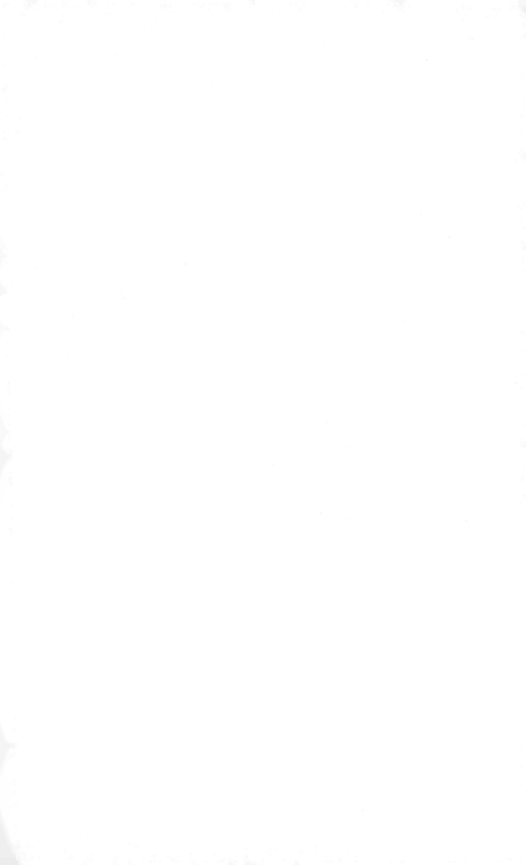

Printed in the United States
130115LV00003B/157/A

9 781932 672558

Certified
Christ-based
Weight Management

▪ When You Are Dying To Eat ▪

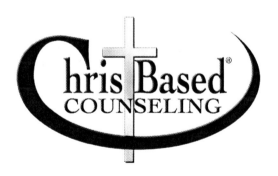

by Dr. Steven B. DavidSon

Outskirts Press, Inc.
Denver, Colorado

Certified Christ-based Weight Management
When You Are Dying To Eat

Biblical references: The Authorized Version of the King James Version is in the public domain.
"Scripture quotations taken from the New American Standard Bible, Copyright 1960, 1962, 1963, 1968, 1971, 1972, 1973, 1975, 1977, 1995 by the Lockman Foundation Used by permission."
(www.Lockman.org)
Scripture quotations marked NLT or New Living Translation are taken from the Holy Bible, New Living Translation, copyright © 1996. Used by permission of Tyndale House Publishers, Inc., Wheaton, Illinois 60189, all rights reserved."

Outskirts Press
http://www.outskirtspress.com

ISBN: 1-932672-55-9

You should consult a physician before beginning any weight loss program.

Outskirts Press and the "OP" logo are trademarks belonging to Outskirts Press, Inc.

Printed in the United States of America